YOUR KNOWLEDGE HAS VALUE

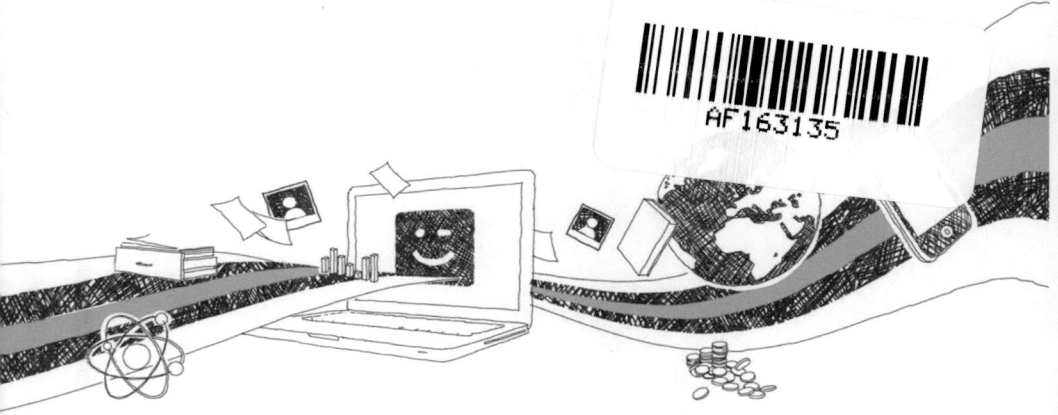

- We will publish your bachelor's and master's thesis, essays and papers

- Your own eBook and book - sold worldwide in all relevant shops

- Earn money with each sale

Upload your text at www.GRIN.com and publish for free

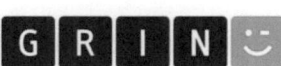

Bibliographic information published by the German National Library:

The German National Library lists this publication in the National Bibliography; detailed bibliographic data are available on the Internet at http://dnb.dnb.de .

This book is copyright material and must not be copied, reproduced, transferred, distributed, leased, licensed or publicly performed or used in any way except as specifically permitted in writing by the publishers, as allowed under the terms and conditions under which it was purchased or as strictly permitted by applicable copyright law. Any unauthorized distribution or use of this text may be a direct infringement of the author s and publisher s rights and those responsible may be liable in law accordingly.

Imprint:

Copyright © 2005 GRIN Verlag
Print and binding: Books on Demand GmbH, Norderstedt Germany
ISBN: 9783668937000

This book at GRIN:

https://www.grin.com/document/471344

Timothy John Whittard

The potential benefits and difficulties associated with interprofessional collaborative working

GRIN Verlag

GRIN - Your knowledge has value

Since its foundation in 1998, GRIN has specialized in publishing academic texts by students, college teachers and other academics as e-book and printed book. The website www.grin.com is an ideal platform for presenting term papers, final papers, scientific essays, dissertations and specialist books.

Visit us on the internet:

http://www.grin.com/

http://www.facebook.com/grincom

http://www.twitter.com/grin_com

Discuss the potential benefits and difficulties associated with interprofessional collaborative working, drawing examples from your own experience of the collaborative group work that forms an integral aspect of the module. (2908 words)

The following essay aims to explore different aspects of interprofessional collaboration across healthcare professions, and highlights the benefits and potential difficulties associated with interprofessional working. These topics were discussed extensively within my interprofessional group, and were investigated through enquiry-based learning. The British Medical Association (2004) states that:

> "Enquiry based learning (EBL) refers to forms of learning driven by a process of enquiry: this usually involves a deep engagement with a complex problem. (...) It can take several forms including analysis, problem solving and research."

The issues that were raised and discussed within my interprofessional group during our enquiry-based learning sessions will form the basis of this assignment. Russell and Hymans (1999) define the term 'interprofessional collaboration' as:

> "Interaction between or among the members of two or more disciplines involving professionals who work together, with intention, mutual respect and commitment for the sake of a more adequate response to a human problem."

Whilst the concept of interprofessional teamwork has been present since the early 1900s (National League for Nursing, 1998), interprofessional education schemes for healthcare professionals only came into existence in the 1960s (Page and Meerabeau, 2004), and it was only in the 1970s that this approach to working was beginning to be incorporated into the field of healthcare (Madge and Khair, 2000). Therefore, one can assume that traditionally, healthcare professionals did not receive much or any interprofessional education or training, and this could explain the difficulties in implementing such methods of working. However, increasingly, over recent years interprofessional working has been considered a crucial aspect of providing efficient and effective holistic healthcare; today it is widely argued that successful interprofessional collaboration increases the "achievement of positive outcomes for service users" (Gair and Hartery, 2001). Headrick et al (1998) highlight the importance of consistency and continuity in utilising an interprofessional approach to healthcare delivery, by stating that virtually everyone receiving healthcare "interacts with more than one health professional"; this reiterates the need for healthcare workers to possess good interprofessional skills. Lax and Galvin (2002) suggest that changes to health and social care policy and the needs of service users have fuelled the increased demand on healthcare professionals to work collaboratively. As patient and client care needs become increasingly complex, successful teamwork between healthcare professionals is needed (Zwarenstein et al, 2005).

The NHS (2002) reports that there is a history of healthcare systems working against one another, and stresses the importance of collaboration across different professions and trusts. This is just one of many new government health policies which stress the importance of interprofessional collaboration "to ensure more integrated health and social care services" (Rolls et al, 2002). The NHS Modernisation Agency (2003) reinforce this by stating that successful teamwork is to be a "key component" of reform within the NHS. In addition to this, Coombs and Dillon (2002) report that in the United Kingdom the government is encouraging widespread modernisation of the working methods and roles of healthcare professionals, with the intention of developing a more effective, patient-centred approach to the delivery of care through teamwork and collaboration between professionals.

There are clearly many benefits of implementing successful interprofessional collaboration, which explains the reasoning behind an increase in government policy advocating interprofessional working and education in the United Kingdom. However, these advantages are not limited to only effecting the patients and clients receiving healthcare, but also benefit the healthcare professionals themselves. Adamson et al (1995) suggest that job satisfaction is linked to interprofessional collaboration; AbuAlRub (2004) reports that effective collaboration and support between colleagues reduces the perception of work-related stress, and this has the potential to improve the quality of treatment for patients through more efficient teamwork and better staff performance. Interprofessional teamwork facilitates bonding and can improve relationships between team members, by allowing the team to learn about one another (Abbott et al, 2005). I was able to experience this for myself during the first enquiry-based learning session for this module. The students that formed the group were a combination of 'adult' student nurses and 'mental health' student nurses; these students had not met one another before. The group was divided into two teams and both teams were immediately set the task of constructing a tower from paper and cardboard, as tall as they possibly could, within a given time. This seemed rather trivial at the time, however it clearly illustrates how interprofessional collaboration helps team members to bond, because although we were all strangers to one another, the teams were able to work together towards a common goal. When the task was completed the groups began mixing and socialising within themselves, suggesting that the teamwork orientated task had facilitated group bonding in both of the two groups. This suggests that good interprofessional practice is advantageous to all parties involved.

It can be argued that interprofessional collaboration is of great support to the individual receiving the healthcare, their carer and also their family, as it can include them all in the decision making processes surrounding the delivery of holistic healthcare, and "focuses" on the entire personal needs of the individual (Headrick et al, 1998). Toop (1998) supports this by suggesting that the shared responsibility over the provision of healthcare in interprofessional teams leads to an improvement in patient-centred care. Therefore, an important step in achieving better patient-centred healthcare is to utilise superior interprofessional teamwork (Kremitske and West, 1997). Mandy et al (2004) reinforce the advantages of interprofessional collaboration, stating that interprofessional teamwork is fundamental in order to provide "optimum healthcare delivery", and according to Roberts and Priest (1997) interprofessional collaboration is essential for "good practice". The quality of healthcare that clients and patients receive is, therefore dependent on the teamwork of the healthcare professionals, which are providing that care (Kaas et al, 2000); this is backed up by Browne and Odell (2004), who state that "skill-mixing" within teams is an essential aspect of good "workforce planning". CAIPE (1996) suggest that this is because "the complexities of care cannot be met by the expertise of any one profession in isolation". When creating a team it is imperative that the individuals within that team possess "personalities and skills" which "compliment" one another, this ensures the presence of "the necessary talent and skill sets to accomplish set goals" (Hill and Ingala, 2001). Therefore good communication among team members is crucial, in order to guarantee that the assortment of "talent and skills" possessed by different members across an interprofessional team are co-ordinated and used effectively to their potential, "so that every patient gets the right care" (NHS, 2000)

Whilst there are clearly numerous advantages to utilising successful interprofessional collaboration, there are also many significant problems in adopting such an approach. There are numerous factors, which have the ability to reduce the success of interprofessional working. Rolls et al (2002) identify three significant inhibitory factors as; "poor communication, conflicting power relations and role confusion". The term 'interprofessional collaboration' and the methods of applying this to clinical practice continue to be areas of poor understanding for healthcare professionals (Kenny, 2002). The confusion and potential problems surrounding working collaboratively are clearly demonstrated in the case of Victoria Climbié; where a "lack of communication and co-ordination" among a range of professional groups failed to prevent an appalling case of child abuse, which eventually led to murder (Royal College of General Practitioners, 2003). The Victoria Climbié case was raised as a topic of discussion during an enquiry-based learning session, and was researched heavily by the group. It became clear through our research and reading surrounding this case that good communication is crucial in order to guarantee effective interprofessional collaboration. Daly (2004) supports this, stating that clear communication between interprofessional team members is an essential "linchpin of successful collaboration". Poor communication between the professionals involved in the Victoria Climbié case was an immense factor in allowing her child abuse to continue unnoticed (The Victoria Climbié Inquiry, 2003), even though there was an abundance of evidence detailing frequent suspicious injuries and incidents, which were not investigated or followed up. The BBC (2003) state that at the public inquiry twelve separate occasions were highlighted where authorities had the opportunity to intervene and prevent further abuse from occurring, but failed to do so.

The sharing of information and communication between members of the interprofessional team was consistently poor in every aspect of this case; for example, the BBC (2003) report that on one occasion social services had been contacted anonymously and informed that Victoria Climbié was "in danger"; the senior social worker involved denied that he or any of his colleagues received information detailing a "potentially serious child protection case". This indicates that a serious communication error took place, which meant that this information was not shared or investigated. Communication difficulties are a significant problem when implementing interprofessional collaboration, and quite obviously these difficulties can have disastrous consequences.

Todd et al (1998) highlight that communication difficulties within teams can lead to "poor group dynamics" and detract from job performance and satisfaction. Roberts and Priest (1997) acknowledge this, and suggest that one cause of communication misunderstanding in an interprofessional setting is the difference in "knowledge base and terminology" used by various professionals. This is supported by Headrick et al (1998) who draw attention to the language variations and "jargon" used by different professional groups, however they also indicate that this is caused by differing educational preparation between professions. Therefore, one possible method for overcoming these differences may be to adopt interprofessional education schemes across healthcare professions "at both pre- and post-qualification levels" (Roberts and Priest, 1997). This would allow the barriers and boundaries between professional groups to be crossed, and enable healthcare workers to develop an understanding of the roles and working practices of other professionals.

Confusion and lack of knowledge regarding the roles and responsibilities of each member within an interprofessional team is another factor, which leads to difficulties in implementing successful interprofessional collaboration, and detracts from the ability of the team to provide good holistic healthcare. Pearson (2003) emphasises the severity of this, stating that both "role confusion and role conflict" are now widespread problems in the field of healthcare. It is, therefore, increasingly necessary for healthcare professionals to have an awareness and knowledge of the roles of other professionals within an interprofessional team; the reasons for this are clearly demonstrated in the Victoria Climbié case. The Victoria Climbié Inquiry (2003) details that after one of her numerous admissions to hospital, although she was deemed medically fit enough to be discharged, the doctor involved felt that "she had yet to provide a satisfactory account of what had happened to her". The doctor then identified that a "proper history" should be obtained, but failed to take any further action, as he wrongly assumed that the nursing staff would do this. Evidently, both the doctor and the nursing staff failed to acquire an account of what had happened to Victoria Climbié, and she was subsequently discharged back into the care of her abusers. This indicates that a gross lack of knowledge regarding the roles of other professional groups led to essential work being omitted, where professionals incorrectly assumed that others would follow up and further investigate the case. Toop (1998) offers one possible explanation for the reason that this crucial work was omitted, claiming that interprofessional teamwork can "blur" the roles and responsibilities of team members, and this can potentially cause a decline in the quality of personal care as this can lead to the duplication or omission of work. Pearson (2003) agrees, stating that the role of the nurse within an interprofessional team has become an area of increasing "ambiguity and debate". Therefore, in order to minimise and prevent "dysfunction" within interprofessional teams, it is an essential requirement that team members have a shared and mutual understanding of the roles of other professionals working within that team (Rowe, 1996). The lack of awareness and knowledge regarding the roles of other professionals, which was demonstrated in the Victoria Climbié case, is again indicative that an increase in interprofessional education is required among healthcare professionals (Department of Health, 2003).

As well as enabling interprofessional team members to acquire a good understanding of the roles of other team members, interprofessional education may also be a useful method of preventing and minimising conflict within interprofessional groups. "Interprofessional rivalry, tribalism and stereotypes" are all types of conflict, which present barriers to successful collaboration within the field of healthcare (Mandy et al, 2004). Roberts and Priest (1997) suggest that interprofessional education offers a solution in overcoming this these barriers, by providing "the opportunity to develop mutual understanding and respect", whilst also recognising "professional difference and expertise".

The Victoria Climbié Inquiry (2003) reports that three different social workers involved in the Victoria Climbié case all testified that they experienced interprofessional conflict. It is reported that one social worker recalled "that there always appeared to be conflict" in the investigation and assessment teams, in which she worked. A second social worker who required a full month of sick leave due to "work-related stress" reported "chronic conflict and tension" among her colleagues and fellow team members; whilst a third social worker, reported that the team in which she worked was "very divided", causing the workplace to feel "hostile"; unsurprisingly, this created a difficult environment in which "to work constructively". Clearly the conflict experienced here had no beneficial effect on the collaborative efforts of the teams involved. Cox (2003) reiterates the difficulties created by conflict between team members and colleagues, stating that conflict within interprofessional groups has "a negative impact on team performance effectiveness". This was demonstrated when I was working as a healthcare assistant on an acute in-patient mental health ward, where the entire nursing team witnessed a heated argument between two members of staff during the nursing handover; this created tension among the team and an uncomfortable working atmosphere.

Dysfunction and conflict within interprofessional collaborative efforts can be caused by a variety of complex factors; however, conflict caused by issues of power and dominance is common. A hierarchy of power within interprofessional collaborative teams creates "strain between professions" (Fagin and Garelick, 2004); Adams and Bond (2000) support this, stating that hierarchies and power struggles in the workplace lead to poor collaboration between professionals and an increase in job dissatisfaction among nursing staff. The hierarchical power struggles experienced within an interprofessional healthcare team are often associated with issues of 'medical dominance'; Gair and Hartery (2001) state that medical dominance lowers the morale of healthcare professionals within an interprofessional team, by causing them to "negatively evaluate their lower status and lack of autonomy relative to doctors". Adamson et al (1995) reinforce this, stating that members of nursing staff, which perceive high levels of medical dominance, possess a low degree of "workplace satisfaction". Medical dominance is attributed to "detracting from the achievement of positive patient outcomes", and therefore a "medically dominated professional hierarchy" is likely to create a reduction in the quality of patient care (Gair and Hartery, 2001). However, Davies (2000) states that "nursing is no more conducive to collaborative working than is medicine" and that change is required within both professions "if a collaborative model is to work".

In conclusion, through my reading around the subject of interprofessional collaboration, and the research carried out in our enquiry-based learning sessions it is clear that successful interprofessional teamwork carries many benefits. Furthermore, advances and improvements in interprofessional education have led to an increase in the implementation of effective collaboration between professionals in clinical practice. However, it is also clear that there is further need for an improvement in interprofessional working. Therefore, this is indicative that more interprofessional education schemes are required in order to eradicate barriers between professional groups.

It is also interesting to note that much of my reading for this module indicated that medical students and doctors are often resistive to interprofessional education schemes (Sheets Cook, 2002), and receive much less interprofessional education in comparison to other healthcare professionals. Page and Meerabeau (2004) explain that medical students were exempt from the first interprofessional education initiatives during the 1960s, whilst professionals in the fields of "nursing; social work; the professions allied to medicine; and complementary therapies" were all included in these interprofessional education schemes. Today, there continues to be only a "few" education programmes, which "involve medical students" (Morison et al, 2003). Roberts and Priest (1997) suggest that these "differences in professional education have helped to maintain boundaries between professional groups", by creating a "professional elitism". Therefore, "educational changes" are still needed, "such as joint sessions between medical and nursing students" (Page and Meerabeau, 2004). Morison et al (2003) state that more opportunities should be provided for medical students to receive interprofessional education, if they are "to acquire team-working skills and to develop an understanding of the functions and roles of other healthcare professionals".

This module has taught me about the importance of interprofessional collaboration, and I feel that I have gained valuable knowledge and skills with regard to working collaboratively which will be of great use to me in the workplace. By working collaboratively throughout this module with 'adult' student nurses, I believe that I have obtained a better understanding and sympathy of the working methods and problems facing this professional group; the understanding created here can only be of benefit to the success of future interprofessional collaboration.

Reference List

Abbott, D., Townsley, R. and Watson, D. (2005) Multi-agency working in services for disabled children: what impact does it have on professionals? *Health and Social Care in the Community* 13(2) 155-163.

AbuAlRub, R.F. (2004) Job Stress, Job Performance, and Social Support Among Hospital Nurses. *Journal of Nursing Scholarship* 36(1) 73–78.

Adams, A. and Bond, S. (2000) Hospital nurses' job satisfaction, individual and organizational characteristics. *Journal or Advanced Nursing* 32(3) 536-543.

Adamson, B.J., Kenny, D.T. and Wilson-Barnett, J. (1995) The impact of perceived medical dominance on the workplace satisfaction of Australian and British nurses. *Journal or Advanced Nursing* 21(1) 172-183.

BBC (2003) Timeline: Victoria Climbié. – [online]. Available from: http://news.bbc.co.uk/1/hi/uk/2062590.stm [Accessed 27th October 2005].

British Medical Association (2004) Enquiry-Based Learning. *Medical education A to Z.* - [online]. Available from: http://www.bma.org.uk/ap.nsf/content/mededatoze [Accessed 16th October 2005].

Browne, A.C. and Odell, M. (2004) A review of nursing skill-mix to optimise care in an acute trust. *Nursing Times* 100(6) 34-38.

CAIPE (1996) *Principles of Interprofessional Education.* CAIPE London.

Coombs, M. and Dillon, A. (2002) Crossing boundaries, re-defining care: the role of the critical care outreach team. *Journal of Clinical Nursing* 11(3) 387-393.

Cox, K.B. (2003) The Effects of Intrapersonal, Intragroup, and Intergroup Conflict on Team Performance Effectiveness and Work Satisfaction. *Nursing Administration Quarterly* 27(2) 153–163.

Daly, G. (2004) Understanding the barriers to multiprofessional collaboration. *Nursing Times* 100(9) 78-79.

Davies, C. (2000) Getting health professionals to work together: There's more to collaboration than simply working side by side. *British Medical Journal* 320(7241) 1021-1022.

Department of Health (2003) *Keeping Children Safe: The Government's Response to the Victoria Climbie Inquiry Report and Joint Chief Inspectors' Report Safeguarding Children*. Crown copyright.

Fagin, L. and Garelick, A. (2004) The doctor–nurse relationship. *Advances in Psychiatric Treatment* (10) 277-286.

Gair, G. and Hartery, T. (2001) Medical dominance in multidisciplinary teamwork: a case study of discharge decision-making in a geriatric assessment unit. *Journal of Nursing Management* 9(1) 3-11.

Headrick, L.A., Wilcock, P.M. and Batalden, P.B. (1998) Continuing medical education: Interprofessional working and continuing medical education. *British Medical Journal* 316(7133) 771-774.

Hill, K. and Ingala, J. (2001) Build a dream team. *Nursing Management* 32(9) 37-38.

Kaas, M.J., Dehn, D., Dahl, D., Frank, K., Markley, J. and Hebert, P. (2000) A View of Prescriptive Practice Collaboration: Perspectives of Psychiatric-Mental Health Clinical Nurse Specialists and Psychiatrists. *Archives of Psychiatric Nursing* 14(5) 222-234.

Kenny, G. (2002) Interprofessional working: opportunities and challenges. *Nursing Standard* 17(6) 33-35.

Kremitske, D. and West, E. (1997) Patient-focused primary care: A model. *Hospital Topics* 75(4) 22–28.

Lax, W. and Galvin, K. (2002) Reflections on a community action research project: interprofessional issues and methodological problems. *Journal of Clinical Nursing* 11(3) 376-386.

Madge, S. and Khair, K. (2000) Multidisciplinary Teams in the United Kingdom: Problems and Solutions. *Journal of Pediatric Nursing* 15(2) 131-134.

Mandy, A., Milton, C. and Mandy, P. (2004) Professional stereotyping and interprofessional education. *Learning in Health and Social Care* 3(3) 154–170.

Morison, S., Boohan, M., Jenkins, J., Moutray, M. (2003) Facilitating undergraduate interprofessional learning in healthcare: comparing classroom and clinical learning for nursing and medical students. *Learning in Health and Social Care* 2(2) 92–104.

National League for Nursing (1998) Building Community: Developing Skills for Interprofessional Health Professions Education and Relationship-Centered Care. *National League for Nursing* 19(2) 86-90.

NHS (2002) *Delivering the NHS Plan – next steps on investment, next steps on reform.* Crown copyright.

NHS Modernisation Agency (2003) *Teamworking for improvement: Planning for spread and sustainability* – [online]. Available from: http://www.modern.nhs.uk/researchintopractice/14993/15038/5th%20(Teamworking).pdf [Accessed 17th October 2005].

Page, S. and Meerabeau, L. (2004) Hierarchies of evidence and hierarchies of education: reflections on a multiprofessional education initiative. *Learning in Health and Social Care* 3(3) 118–128.

Pearson, A. (2003) Multidisciplinary nursing: re-thinking role boundaries. *Journal of Clinical Nursing* 12(5) 625–629.

Roberts, P. and Priest, H. (1997) Achieving interprofessional working in mental health. *Nursing Standard* 12(2) 39-41.

Rolls, L., Davis, E. and Coupland, K. (2002) Improving serious mental illness through interprofessional education. *Journal of Psychiatric and Mental Health Nursing* 9(3) 317–324.

Rowe, H. (1996) Multidisciplinary teamwork - myth or reality? *Journal of Nursing Management* 4(2) 93-101.

Royal College of General Practitioners (2003) *The Victoria Climbié Inquiry Report. Sixth Report of the House of Commons Health Committee Session 2002-3.* Summary Paper.

Russell, K.M. and Hymans, D. (1999) Interprofessional Education for Undergraduate Students. *Public Health Nursing* 16(4) 254-262.

Sheets Cook, S. (2002) Evaluating the merits of interdisciplinary education. *Nursing Times* 98(41) 30-32.

Todd, C.J., Farquhar, M.C. and Camilleri-Ferrante, C. (1998) Team midwifery: the views and job satisfaction of midwives. *Midwifery* (14) 214-224.

Toop, L. (1998) Primary care: core values: Patient centred primary care. *British Medical Journal* 316(7148) 1882-1883.

The Victoria Climbié Inquiry (2003). Crown copyright.

Zwarenstein, M., Reeves, S., Barr, H., Hammick, M., Koppel, I. and Atkins, J. (2005) Interprofessional education: effects on professional practice and health care outcomes. *The Cochrane Database of Systematic Reviews* (4). The Cochrane Library, Copyright.

YOUR KNOWLEDGE HAS VALUE

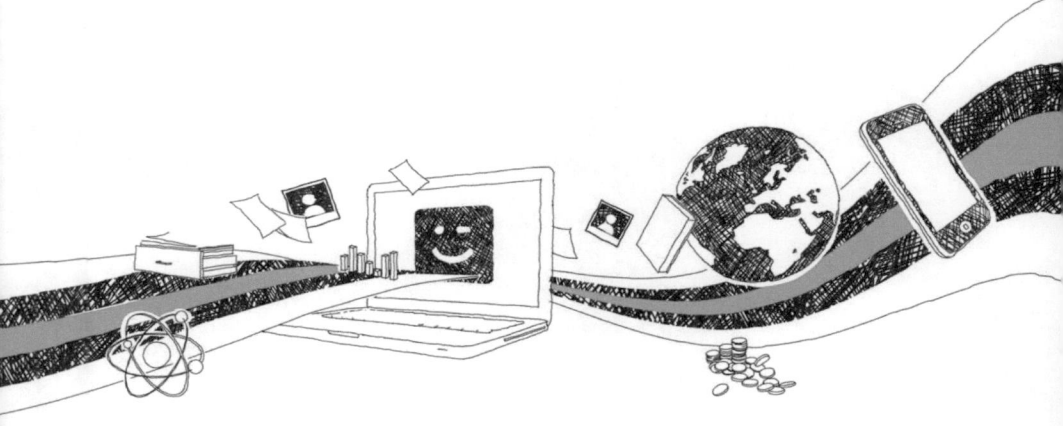

- We will publish your bachelor's and master's thesis, essays and papers

- Your own eBook and book - sold worldwide in all relevant shops

- Earn money with each sale

Upload your text at www.GRIN.com and publish for free

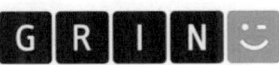